THE BONE CANCER DIET COOKBOOK

Recipes That Promote a Healthy Diet and Speed the Recovery Process from Bone Cancer

REX LEWIS

Table of Contents

Introduction

For those who have been diagnosed with bone cancer, it is imperative to maintain a healthy, balanced diet. A healthy body is better equipped to handle the difficulties of cancer therapy, promote general health, and facilitate the healing process. There isn't a special "bone cancer diet," although patients receiving therapy may benefit from several dietary considerations. It's crucial to remember that dietary suggestions can change depending on a person's unique medical condition, course of treatment, and nutritional requirements.

Important Elements of a Diet for Bone Cancer:

1. Sufficient Consumption of Protein:

• Protein is necessary for bone regrowth and tissue healing.

• Fish, poultry, beans, lentils, tofu, and dairy products are sources of lean protein.

2. Nutrient-Rich Foods: To acquire important vitamins, minerals, and antioxidants, eat a range of fruits and vegetables.

• Colorful foods, veggies, and dark leafy greens are good for your general health.

3. Calcium and Vitamin D: Sufficient consumption of these nutrients is essential for healthy bones.

• Leafy greens, dairy products, sun exposure, and fortified plant-based milk are good sources.

4. Hydration: It's critical to maintain adequate hydration, particularly while receiving cancer therapy.

• Fruit juices that has been diluted, herbal teas, and water can all aid in keeping you hydrated.

5. Balanced Carbohydrates: To gain long-lasting energy, choose whole grains, legumes, and vegetables.

• Restrict the amount of refined and processed carbs.

6. Healthy Fats: Add foods like avocados, almonds, seeds, and olive oil that are rich in healthy fats.

• Fatty fish, such as salmon, contain omega-3 fatty acids, which may have anti-inflammatory effects.

7. Reduce Processed Food Intake:
Cut back on processed and sugary foods since they may worsen general health and cause inflammation.

8. Smaller, More Often Meals:
Consuming smaller, more regular meals might help control hunger and ease gastrointestinal pain.

Personalized Dietary Advice:
Speak with a qualified dietitian or nutritionist for advice on a customized diet based on your unique nutritional requirements, treatment side effects, and medical conditions.

Things to Think About During Treatment:

• Certain cancer treatments can have adverse effects on taste, appetite, or digestion. It's critical to modify the diet to account for these modifications.

• Common objectives during cancer therapy include preventing malnutrition, controlling nausea, and maintaining weight.

Open communication is vital to addressing any unique dietary issues or limits connected to an individual's treatment plan with the healthcare team.

In the end, a healthy, nutrient-rich diet can improve general wellbeing and help the body cope with the difficulties of treating bone cancer. Seek counsel from medical specialists for specific recommendations and direction at all times.

CHAPTER ONE
Knowing About Bone Cancer

Recognizing the many forms, causes, symptoms, diagnosis, and available treatments is essential to understanding bone cancer. Here's a detailed rundown:

1. Bone cancer types:

• **Primary Bone Cancer:** Develops in the bones initially.

• **Osteosarcoma:** Usually affects lengthy bones, common in teenagers.

• **Chondrosarcoma**: A common adult condition that develops in cartilage.

Children and young adults can be affected by Ewing sarcoma.

• Metastatic (secondary) bone cancer: This type of cancer starts elsewhere in the body and progresses to the bones.

2. Causes and Risk Factors: It's not always clear what causes what.

• The risk may be raised by radiation exposure, genetic factors, and certain inherited disorders.

• Metastasis from other primary tumors causes secondary bone cancer.

3. Symptoms: ongoing discomfort in the bones.

• A bump or swelling on the bone.

• Exhaustion and weakness.

• Breaks brought on by weakening bones.

• Loss of weight without cause.

4. Diagnosis:

• **Imaging Tests:** to visualize abnormalities, X-rays, CT, MRI, and bone scans are performed.

• **Biopsy:** The removal of tissue for microscopic inspection in order to diagnose malignancy.

- **Blood Tests:** Evaluating certain indicators that might point to bone cancer.

5. Staging: Ascertains the degree and dispersal of the cancer.

- Stages vary from IV (advanced with metastases) to I (localized).

6. Course of Treatment: Excision of the tumor or damaged bone, occasionally with repair.

- **Chemotherapy:** Medication to eradicate or inhibit the spread of cancer cells.

• **Radiation therapy:** Cancer cells are targeted by high-energy radiation.

• **Targeted therapy:** Drugs that specifically target molecules implicated in the development of cancer.

• **Immunotherapy:** To combat cancer, it strengthens the immune system.

7. Prognosis: Varying according on cancer kind, stage, and response to treatment.

• Treatment and early detection lead to better results.

• The prognosis for metastatic bone cancer is typically less good.

8. Supportive Care: Physical therapy, psychological counseling, and pain control.

• Nutritional help to sustain vitality and strength while undergoing therapy.

9. Follow-Up: Consistently keeping an eye out for recurrences and overseeing the treatment's long-term consequences.

10. Clinical Trials: Taking part in clinical trials may provide access to cutting-edge medical interventions.

11. Survivorship: Pay attention to the physical and emotional elements of post-treatment well-being.

Collaborating closely with a multidisciplinary healthcare team of oncologists, surgeons, radiologists, and supportive care workers is crucial for persons diagnosed with bone cancer. A comprehensive approach to controlling bone cancer includes open communication, routine screenings, and commitment to the treatment plan.

Bone Cancer Types

Primary bone cancer and secondary (metastatic) bone cancer are two categories for bone cancer. Whereas secondary bone cancer develops when cancer from other parts of the body spreads to the bones, primary bone cancer starts in the bones.

Primary Cancer of the Bones:

Osteosarcoma: The most prevalent type of primary bone cancer.

• Frequently affects long bones, including the arms and legs.

• Often diagnosed in young adults and teenagers.

• A tumor with an aggressive growth pattern.

2. Chondrosarcoma: This cancer starts in the cartilage cells.

• Affects adults primarily.

• Usually located in the arms, legs, and pelvis.

• Grows often more slowly than osteosarcoma.

3. Ewing Sarcoma: Affects mostly youth and young adults.

• Frequently develops in the arms, legs, or pelvic bones.

• Defined by spherical, tiny cells.

• Has a propensity for aggression and metastasis.

4. Chordoma: Rare tumor typically found in the base of the skull or the spine.

• Is formed from the remains of the notochord, a structure that exists throughout fetal growth.

• Slow-growing but frequently invasive in certain areas.

5. Fibrosarcoma: An uncommon kind of bone cancer.

• Develops from the bone's fibrous tissue.

• Can happen in any bone, although the arms and legs are the most typical places to find it.

Secondary (Metastatic) Bone Cancer

This type of bone cancer develops when cancer cells go to the bones from other places of the body. The following are typical primary malignancies that could spread to the bones:

1. Breast Cancer: Advanced breast cancer frequently metastasizes to the bones.

2. Lung Cancer: The spine and pelvis are the two main places where lung cancer can spread to bones.

3. Prostate Cancer: The hips and spine are the most prevalent places when prostate cancer metastasizes.

4. Kidney Cancer: Secondary bone tumors can result from the spread of kidney cancer to the bones.

5. Thyroid Cancer: The spine is especially vulnerable to thyroid cancer metastases.

6. Multiple Myeloma: A kind of blood cancer that mostly affects bone marrow plasma cells.

- Causes malignancies to grow inside the bones.

Determining the right course of treatment requires an understanding of the type of bone cancer. Plans for treatment are frequently customized based on the unique features of the cancer, such as its kind, stage, and location. Better results can be achieved by early detection and a multidisciplinary strategy that includes supportive care, radiation therapy, chemotherapy, and surgery.

Reasons and Danger Elements

Although the precise origins of primary bone cancer are frequently unknown, a number of risk factors may make the disease more likely to occur. It's crucial to remember that the presence of one or more risk factors does not ensure the development of bone cancer; those without known risk factors may still be impacted. **The following are some typical causes and risk factors for bone cancer:**

Primary Bone Cancer Risk Factors:

1. Age: Adolescents and young adults are frequently affected by osteosarcoma, the most prevalent kind of primary bone cancer.

• In adults, chondrosarcoma is more prevalent.

2. Gender: Chondrosarcoma affects both sexes equally, although osteosarcoma is significantly more common in men.

3. Genetic Factors: Hereditary retinoblastoma and Li-Fraumeni syndrome are two genetic disorders that may raise the risk of bone cancer.

4. Radiation Exposure: Prior exposure to high radiation doses, whether as a result of medical treatment or for other purposes, may raise the chance of developing bone cancer.

5. Paget's Disease: Osteosarcoma is more likely to occur in people with Paget's disease of the bone.

6. Bone Marrow Diseases: Bone marrow-related conditions, such as myelodysplastic syndromes, may be linked to a higher risk.

7. Metallic Implants: Research points to a possible connection between the emergence of bone cancer and metallic implants, such as joint replacements. The total danger is minimal, though.

Risk elements for metastatic (secondary) bone cancer:

1. Primary Cancer Diagnosis: Those who have been diagnosed with a primary cancer, particularly those of the breast, lung, prostate, kidney, or thyroid, are more likely to experience metastases that result in secondary bone cancer.

2. Age: Although metastatic bone cancer can strike anyone at any age, the risk rises with advancing years.

3. Advanced Cancer Stage: Primary cancers with an increased propensity to spread to the bones are those in advanced stages.

4. Use of some Medications: The chance of developing bone metastases may increase with the use of some chemotherapy medications, among other cancer treatments.

5. Weaker Immune System: People who take certain medications or have illnesses like

HIV/AIDS may have a weaker immune system, which makes them more vulnerable to metastatic bone cancer.

It is crucial to comprehend these risk factors in order to diagnose and treat them early. For those who are at risk or have been diagnosed with bone cancer, improved results can be achieved by routine medical check-ups, early diagnosis, and proper treatment. For individualized evaluations and advice, people should speak with healthcare providers if they have concerns about their risk of developing bone cancer.

CHAPTER TWO
Signs and Prognosis

Signs of cancer of the bone:

1. Persistent Bone ache: The most typical symptom is a persistent, often worsening ache in a particular bone.

2. Lump or Swelling: The formation of a lump on or close to the injured bone.

3. Weakened Bones: Even with small injuries, cancer-weakened bones might result in fractures.

4. Fatigue: Severe weakness or weariness that may go hand in hand with advanced bone cancer.

5. Unexplained Weight Loss: Notable cause for a notable drop in weight.

6. Joint Stiffness: Restricted mobility or stiffness in joints close to the damaged bone.

7. Fever: A low-grade fever has been linked in certain instances to bone cancer.

8. Night Sweats: Prolonged perspiration at night.

It's crucial to remember that these symptoms are not always indicative of bone cancer and can possibly be linked to a number of other illnesses. Nonetheless, a medical expert should be consulted if symptoms are severe or persistent.

Identification of Bone Cancer:

1. Medical History and Physical Examination: In addition to performing a physical examination, the healthcare professional will inquire about the patient's symptoms and medical history.

2. Imaging Examinations:

• X-rays: To see the bones and spot any irregularities.

• **CT Scan:** Offers precise cross-sectional pictures of the skeleton.

• **MRI:** Provides detailed pictures of the soft tissues surrounding bones.

• **Bone Scan:** Assists in locating anomalous bone activity.

3. Biopsy: A biopsy is used to get a conclusive diagnosis of bone cancer.

• A tiny sample of the questionable tissue is taken out and examined under a microscope.

• Two types of biopsies are surgical and needle biopsies.

4. Blood Tests: The presence of bone cancer may result in higher values of several blood tests, such as alkaline phosphatase.

It is possible to evaluate additional blood indicators based on the type of bone cancer that is suspected.

5. Bone Marrow Examination: To determine whether the bone marrow is affected by malignancy, a bone marrow biopsy may be necessary in certain circumstances.

6. Imaging for Staging: Following a diagnosis, other imaging tests, like PET scans or chest X-rays, may be carried out to ascertain the cancer's extent, or stage.

7. Genetic Testing: Genetic testing might be advised in certain circumstances, particularly if there is a possibility that inherited disorders are linked to bone cancer.

8. Consultation with Specialists: To choose the best course of action, orthopedic surgeons, oncologists, and other specialists may need to be consulted, depending on the kind and stage of bone cancer.

A prompt and precise diagnosis is essential to creating a successful treatment strategy. People should seek immediate medical assistance for a comprehensive evaluation by healthcare professionals if they suspect bone cancer.

Dietary Influence on Bone Cancer

For those with a diagnosis of bone cancer, nutrition is essential. A healthy, well-balanced diet can improve general health, assist in reducing the negative effects of treatment, and strengthen the body's defenses against bone cancer. The following are some important things to think about while evaluating how diet affects bone cancer:

1. Sustaining Nutritional State:

• Nutrition absorption, metabolism, and appetite can all be impacted by cancer and its therapies.

• Consuming enough calories, protein, vitamins, and minerals is necessary to maintain general health and prevent malnutrition.

2. Consumption of Proteins in Tissue Repair:

• After surgery or other cancer treatments, protein is especially important for tissue regeneration and repair.

• Lean meats, chicken, fish, dairy products, lentils, and tofu are good sources of protein.

3. Vitamin D and Calcium for Healthy Bones:

• Enough calcium and vitamin D consumption is necessary to keep bones healthy.

• Sources of calcium and vitamin D include dairy products, fortified plant-based milk, leafy greens, and sunshine exposure.

4. Drinking Plenty of Water

• Maintaining adequate hydration is crucial during cancer treatment, as it can aid in the management of adverse symptoms including fatigue and nausea.

• Fruit juices that has been diluted, herbal teas, and water can all help you stay hydrated.

5. Rich in Antioxidants Foods:

• Fruits and vegetables include antioxidants that may help fight oxidative stress brought on by cancer and its therapies.

• Rich in antioxidants include colorful fruits and vegetables, like citrus fruits, berries, and leafy greens.

6. The Fatty Acids Omega-3:

• Walnuts, flaxseeds, and fatty fish like salmon are good sources of omega-3 fatty acids, which may have anti-inflammatory qualities.

• Eating these foods can promote general health and aid in the management of inflammation.

7. Little, Regular Meals:

• Eating more often and in smaller portions may help control hunger and avoid nausea.

• By using this strategy, people can achieve their nutritional goals without overtaxing their digestive systems.

8. Getting Used to Side Effects of Treatment:

• Taste, digestion, and appetite can all be adversely affected by certain cancer treatments.

• It's crucial to adjust the diet to account for these modifications, such as choosing softer or colder foods when mouth sores are present.

9. Customized Food Programs:

• Consulting a nutritionist or licensed dietitian is essential for developing individualized food regimens.

• Taking care of certain dietary requirements, controlling side effects from medication, and maintaining a balanced diet all contribute to general wellbeing.

10. Add-ons as Required:

• Supplements could be suggested in some circumstances to treat particular nutrient shortages.

Supplements, however, are to be used only under a doctor's supervision.

Working together with their healthcare team, which includes dietitians and oncologists, is crucial for people with bone cancer to address their specific dietary needs and create a strategy that promotes general health both before and after treatment. Throughout the course of a cancer diagnosis, regular communication with medical specialists can assist address any issues and maximize nutritional support.

CHAPTER THREE
The Role of Diet in Treating Bone Cancer

When it comes to overall health, the efficacy of treatment and recovery from bone cancer, nutrition is critical. Here's why diet matters when receiving treatment for bone cancer:

1. Assistance for General Health:

• Healthy eating promotes general health in patients receiving therapy for bone cancer.

• Essential nutrients required for immune system function, wound healing, and tissue repair are found in a well-balanced diet.

2. Sustaining Max Power and Vitality:

• Physically taxing cancer therapies like radiation therapy, chemotherapy, and surgery can cause weakness and exhaustion.

• Sufficient nourishment keeps people strong and energized, which make it easier for them to withstand and recover from medical interventions.

3. Increased Tolerance to Treatment:

• Eating a healthy diet can increase treatment tolerance and lower the chance of treatment delays or interruptions.

• Foods high in nutrients help the body cope with the side effects of cancer treatments, like nausea, vomiting, and weight loss.

4. Maintaining Lean Body Mass:

• Why Maintaining lean body mass throughout cancer therapy requires consuming enough protein.

• Treatment results, quality of life, and functional status can all be enhanced by maintaining muscle mass.

5. Encouragement of Bone Health:

• Vitamin D and calcium are essential for healthy bones, and this is particularly true for those who have bone cancer.

• Maintaining bone strength and density with proper nutrition may help lower the incidence of skeletal problems and fractures.

6. Handling Adverse Reactions to Treatment:

• Nutrition can help control treatment-related adverse effects include mouth sores, nausea, and taste alterations.

• Eating softer foods or eating smaller, more frequent meals are two dietary changes that might help reduce pain and increase nutrient intake.

7. Support for the Immune System:

• A healthy diet boosts immunity, which is critical for warding off infections and encouraging recovery during the course of treating bone cancer.

• Foods high in nutrients offer vital vitamins, minerals, and antioxidants that boost immune function.

8. Supporting Recuperation and Rehabilitation:

• After receiving treatment for bone cancer, adequate diet plays a role in the patient's recuperation and rehabilitation.

• Foods high in nutrients promote wound healing, tissue repair, and physical function restoration, all of which improve general quality of life.

9. Malnutrition Prevention:

• The prognosis and results of treatment might be adversely affected by malnutrition, which is prevalent in cancer patients.

• By preventing malnutrition and the problems it causes, nutritional support improves patient outcomes and treatment efficacy.

10. Tailored Assistance:

• Individual requirements should be taken into consideration when making nutrition recommendations, and this includes treatment type, side effects, dietary choices, and nutritional status.

• Working with a certified dietitian or nutritionist can assist people in creating individualized nutrition regimens that address their unique requirements and objectives.

In conclusion, healthy eating is critical to the support of patients receiving therapy for bone cancer. Nutrition plays a vital role in preserving health, bolstering the efficacy of treatment, and improving general quality of life both during and after cancer treatment by giving the body the nutrients it needs.

The Impact of Diet on Bone Health

An essential component of preserving bone health throughout life is nutrition. The vital elements required for bone development, remodeling, and overall skeletal integrity are supplied by a healthy diet. This is how diet impacts the health of bones:

1. Calcium

• **Function:** Calcium is an essential mineral needed for the development and upkeep of bone tissue.

- **Impact:** Inadequate calcium consumption raises the risk of fractures and results in decreased bone mineral density.

- **Sources:** Certain nuts and seeds, fortified plant-based milk, leafy green vegetables, and dairy products.

2. Vitamin D

- **Function:** In order to promote bone mineralization, vitamin D is necessary for the absorption of calcium and phosphorus.

• **Impact:** Inadequate nutrition can weaken bones, which exacerbates diseases like osteoporosis.

• **Sources:** Vitamin D supplements, fatty fish, sun exposure, and fortified foods.

3. Phosphorus:

• **Function:** Another mineral that combines with calcium to build the mineralized structure of bones is phosphorus.

• **Effect:** Preserves bone density and strength.

• **Sources:** Whole grains, meat, fish, poultry, and dairy products.

4. The Mineral Magnesium

• **Function:** Magnesium aids in the conversion of vitamin D to its active form and plays a role in bone mineralization.

• **Effect:** A deficiency may have an impact on bone health and raise the possibility of osteoporosis.

• **Sources:** Legumes, nuts, seeds, whole grains, and leafy green vegetables.

5. Vitamin K:

• **Function:** Proteins involved in bone mineralization and bone metabolism depend on vitamin K.

- **Impact:** Impaired bone mineralization may be a result of deficiency.

- **Sources:** Broccoli, Brussels sprouts, leafy green vegetables, and some vegetable oils.

6. Protein

- **Function:** Protein serves as a building block for bone tissue, enhancing the density and strength of bones.

- **Impact:** Consuming insufficient amounts of protein can harm bones and raise the chance of fractures.

- **Sources:** Plant-based protein sources, dairy products, fish, poultry, and lean meats.

7. Collagen

- **Function:** Collagen gives bones their structural integrity and adds to their strength and flexibility.

- **Impact:** Vitamin C has an impact on collagen formation, and vitamin C is essential for maintaining bone health overall.

- **Sources:** Strawberries, bell peppers, citrus fruits, and other fruits and vegetables.

8. The Fatty Acids Omega-3:

• **Function:** Anti-inflammatory properties of omega-3 fatty acids may promote bone health.

• **Impact:** Studies indicate that consuming omega-3 fatty acids and bone mineral density are positively correlated.

• **Sources:** walnuts, chia seeds, flaxseeds, and fatty fish (such as mackerel and salmon).

9. Restricting Specific Substances:

• **Calcium Inhibitors:** High intakes of certain fibers and excessive caffeine can both affect how well calcium is absorbed.

• **Phosphorus Imbalance:** Bone health may be impacted by an extremely high phosphorus consumption in comparison to calcium.

10. Sustaining a Proper Weight:

• **Role:** Overall bone health depends on maintaining a healthy weight through a balanced diet and frequent exercise.

• **Impact:** Losing too much weight or being underweight raises the possibility of fractures and bone loss.

11. Sufficient Hydration:

• **Function:** Drinking enough water promotes good health in general, including bone health.

• **Impact:** Bone mineral density may be compromised by dehydration.

Balanced, nutrient-rich diets along with a healthy lifestyle go a long way toward maintaining good bone health. It is important to get these nutrients from a range of foods and, if needed, supplements under medical specialists' supervision. Strong and resilient bones are also further promoted by weight-bearing activities and other healthy lifestyle choices.

Laying the Groundwork: Essentials of a Bone-Healthy Diet

Including essential nutrients that support bone health is part of laying the groundwork for a diet that promotes bone health. What constitutes a bone-healthy diet is as follows:

1. Foods High in Calcium:

• **Sources:** Leafy green vegetables (kale, broccoli), dairy products (milk, yogurt, cheese), fortified plant-based milk (soy, almond, oat), and tinned fish with bones (salmon, sardines).

2. Sources of Vitamin D:

• **Sources:** exposure to sunlight, egg yolks, fatty fish (tuna, salmon, and mackerel), and fortified meals (cereals, some dairy products, and plant-based milk).

3. High in Protein Foods:

• Protein sources from plants, such as quinoa, nuts, and seeds, as well as lean meats like chicken and turkey, fish, dairy products, eggs, and legumes like beans and lentils.

4. Complete Grains:

- **Sources:** whole-grain bread and cereals, brown rice, quinoa, whole wheat, and oats.

5. Produce and Fruits:

- **Sources:** Colorful fruits and vegetables are a great way to receive important minerals, vitamins, and antioxidants. For a varied nutrient intake, aim for a rainbow of choices.

6. Rich in Magnesium Foods:

- Nuts (almonds, cashews), seeds (sunflower, pumpkin), whole grains, leafy greens (kale, spinach), and legumes are some of the sources.

7. Foods Containing Vitamin K:

- **Sources:** Brussels sprouts, leafy greens (kale, spinach, broccoli), and some vegetable oils.

8. The Fatty Acids Omega-3:

- **Sources:** Algae-based supplements, walnuts, chia seeds, flaxseeds, and fatty fish (trout, mackerel, salmon).

9. Reducing Sodium and Caffeine:

- Moderation can assist maintain bone health by reducing excessive caffeine intake and regulating sodium intake.

10. Drinking Plenty of Water

• **Significance:** Maintaining adequate hydration is crucial for good general health, which includes strong bones.

• **Sources:** herbal teas, water, and other drinks without caffeine.

11. Sustaining a Proper Weight:

• **Significance:** It's imperative for bone health to attain and sustain a healthy weight via a well-balanced diet and consistent exercise.

- **Balanced Approach:** Steer clear of severe weight loss or underweight situations as they may exacerbate bone loss.

12. Frequent Exercise:

- Exercises involving weight bearing, such as walking, running, dancing, and resistance training, are beneficial for preserving bone density and strength.

13. Exposure to Sunlight:

- **Vitamin D Synthesis:** The body synthesizes vitamin D in part through modest sun exposure.

• **Caution:** To avoid damaging your skin, wear sunscreen.

14. Moderate Intake of Alcohol:

• **Limitation:** If you drink alcohol, use it sparingly because too much of it can harm your bones.

15. Steer Clear Of Smoking:

• **Impact:** Since smoking is linked to a reduction in bone density, giving up smoking or abstaining from it promotes bone health.

16. Consultation with Medical Specialists:

• **Individualized Guidance:** For tailored advice based on specific health requirements, circumstances, and preferences, speak with a licensed dietitian or other healthcare provider.

Strong and durable bones are the result of a healthy lifestyle combined with a well-balanced, nutrient-dense, and diverse diet. Osteoporosis and other disorders affecting the bones can be avoided by maintaining a balance of these dietary components and implementing other bone-friendly practices. Since dietary requirements might differ from person to person, consulting a healthcare provider is advised for specific recommendations.

CHAPTER FOUR
Creating a Diet Plan with a Bone Cancer Focus

Creating a diet plan specifically targeted at bone cancer entails including foods high in nutrients that promote general health and specifically meet the nutritional requirements linked to the disease. It's crucial to remember that each person should have a customized food plan based on their unique needs, stage of treatment, and preferences. The following is a general guide to developing a diet plan targeted at bone cancer:

1. Sufficient Intake of Protein:

• **Sources:** Plant-based protein sources (quinoa, nuts, seeds), dairy products, eggs, legumes (beans, lentils), tofu, and lean meats (turkey, chicken, fish).

• **Significance:** Protein facilitates tissue restoration, which is essential both during and following cancer therapies.

2. Foods High in Calcium and Vitamin D:

• **Sources:** Bony, high-fat fish (salmon, sardines), leafy green vegetables (kale, broccoli), fortified plant-based milk, and dairy products.

• **Significance:** Calcium and vitamin D are vital for healthy bones; they promote treatment results by preserving bone density.

3. The Fatty Acids Omega-3:

• **Sources:** Algae-based supplements, walnuts, chia seeds, flaxseeds, and fatty fish (mackerel, salmon).

• **Importance:** During cancer treatment, omega-3 fatty acids may have anti-inflammatory properties that are advantageous.

4. Produce and Fruits:

• **Sources:** An assortment of vibrant fruits and vegetables that offer vital antioxidants, vitamins, and minerals.

• **Significance:** Promotes immune system performance, general health, and intestinal health by supplying fiber.

5. Complete Grains:

• **Sources:** whole-grain bread and cereals, brown rice, quinoa, whole wheat, and oats.

• **Significance:** Fiber and a variety of nutrients from whole grains support digestive health and energy production.

6. Moderate Energy Consumption:

• **Balance:** To promote general health and stave off weight loss, maintain a balance between calorie intake and energy expenditure.

7. Drinking plenty of water

• **Sources:** herbal teas, water, and other drinks without caffeine.

• **Significance:** Maintaining adequate hydration promotes general health and aids in the management of therapeutic adverse effects.

8. Reducing Sodium and Caffeine:

• **Moderation:** Restrict excessive coffee consumption and consume sodium in moderation.

• **Significance:** Aids in controlling adverse effects of treatment and promotes general well-being.

9. Tailored Food and Nutrition Advice:

• **Consultation:** For individualized guidance based on specific medical problems, treatment regimens, and dietary preferences, speak with a licensed dietitian or nutritionist.

10. Taking Treatment Side Effects into Account:

• **Texture Modifications:** Adjust textures in accordance with side effects of treatment; for example, if you're having trouble swallowing, go for softer foods.

• **Temperature Considerations:** Modify the temperature according to personal preferences and sensitivity levels (for example, serve cold food if you have mouth sores).

11. Frequent Inspections and Modifications:

• **Follow-Up:** Keep a close eye on your nutritional status and modify your meal plan as necessary in response to evolving requirements, treatment outcomes, and general health.

12. Add-ons as Required:

• **Consultation:** With the advice of medical specialists, take into consideration supplements if there are particular nutrient shortages or difficulties satisfying nutritional demands with food alone.

13. Stressing General Well-Being

- **Physical Activity:** To enhance general wellbeing and energy levels, promote modest physical activity when suitable.

14. Psychosocial Assistance:

- Holistic Approach: Take into account the emotional and mental components of nutrition during cancer treatment and include psychosocial assistance.

15. Interaction with the medical staff:

- **Have an Open Dialogue:** Share any worries, side effects, or adjustments to dietary requirements with the medical staff.

A food plan for a person with bone cancer should always take their specific demands and preferences into consideration. Maintaining regular contact with medical experts guarantees that the treatment plan is appropriately tailored to the unique needs and obstacles of the patient.

Foods to Consume If You Have Bone Cancer

Focusing on nutrient-dense foods that promote general health, supply vital nutrients for bone strength, and assist in managing treatment side effects is crucial when creating a diet plan for bone cancer. The following foods should be a part of a diet for bone cancer:

1. Foods High in Protein: Lean Meats (Fish, Turkey, Chicken) Dairy Products (Yogurt, Cheese, Milk) Eggs

- **Beans and lentils;** tofu and other soy-based products;

• Seeds and nuts

• Nut butter (almond and peanut butter)

2. Sources of calcium: Dairy products (milk, yogurt, cheese); Plant-based milk (soy, almond, oat); Broccoli, spinach, and kale; Salmon and sardines in cans; Cereals; and fortified foods (orange juice).

3. Foods High in Vitamin D:

• Omega-3 Fish (tuna, salmon, and mackerel)

• Egg yolks

• Foods fortified with nutrients (cereals, plant-based milk, some dairy products)

4. Sources of Omega-3 Fatty Acids:

walnuts; flaxseeds and flaxseed oil; fatty fish (salmon, mackerel, trout); chia seeds; walnuts; algae-based supplements

5. Foods High in Vitamin K:

• Broccoli; cabbage; collard greens; kale, spinach, and collard greens; • Certain vegetable oils (canola and olive oils)

6. Foods High in Magnesium:

• Nuts and Seeds (Pumpkin, Cashew, and Almond)

• Leafy greens (spinach, Swiss chard);

• Whole grains (brown rice, quinoa, oats);

• Legumes (black beans, chickpeas)

7. Fruits and Vegetables Rich in Antioxidants:

• Citrus fruits (grapefruit, orange, bell peppers)

• Berries (strawberries, blueberries, raspberries)

• Dark leafy greens (kale, spinach)

8. Whole Grains: Quinoa, Barley, Brown Rice, Whole Wheat, and Oats

9. Sources of Hydration: Water; Herbal Teas; Infused Water (including cucumber, lemon, and mint); Coconut Water (which is a natural supply of electrolytes)

10. Foods High in Fiber:

• Whole grains;

• Fruits (bananas, pears, and apples)

• Nuts and seeds;

• Legumes (beans, lentils);

- Vegetables (carrots, broccoli, cauliflower)

11. Iron- and vitamin-C-Rich Foods:

- Foods high in iron include lean meats, chicken, fish, beans, lentils, and fortified cereals.

- Foods high in vitamin C include bell peppers, tomatoes, strawberries, kiwis, and citrus fruits.

12. Foods That Are Easy to Digest for Nausea and Digestive Problems:

Boiled potatoes; rice; toasted bread or crackers; boiled applesauce; cooked fruits (canned peaches, applesauce)

13. Foods Rich in Probiotics and Prebiotics for Gut Health:

• Foods high in prebiotics include bananas, asparagus, leeks, onions, and oats.

• Foods high in probiotics: miso, yogurt, kefir, sauerkraut, and kimchi

14. Foods to Sustain Energy and Weight:

• Rich in nutrients shakes or smoothies made with fruits, veggies, and protein powder

• Nuts, seeds, avocado, olive oil, and other healthy fats; • Regular, small meals and snacks to sustain energy levels;

15. Consulting with Medical Specialists:

•For customized nutritional advice catered to specific requirements, treatment regimens, and dietary preferences, always seek the advice of a qualified dietitian or nutritionist.

During the course of treating bone cancer, a diet rich in these nutrient-dense foods can help maintain bone health, control side effects, and enhance general wellbeing.

CHAPTER FIVE
Fruits and Vegetables that Provide Bone-Building Minerals

Incorporating fruits and vegetables high in nutrients that promote bone health is crucial for maintaining bone health. Numerous vitamins, minerals, and antioxidants found in these meals support strong bones and general health. The following foods and vegetables have elements that strengthen bones:

Fruits:

1. Berries:

Nutrients: Vitamin C, manganese, and antioxidants found in berries—

such as blueberries, strawberries, and raspberries—support collagen synthesis and bone health.

2. Citrus Fruits:

Nutrients: Vitamin C, which is essential for collagen production and bone building, may be found in abundance in oranges, grapefruits, lemons, and limes.

3. Kiwi:

Nutrient-dense: Rich in potassium, vitamin K, and vitamin C, kiwis support strong bones and a robust immune system.

4. Bananas:

Nutrients: Potassium, which is found in bananas, supports bone health and helps the body manage calcium levels.

5. Apples:

Nutrients: Apples are a good source of boron, a trace mineral linked to healthy bones. They also supply fiber and vitamin C.

6. Pineapple:

Nutrients: Vitamin C and manganese in pineapples promote the formation of collagen and the health of bones.

7. Papaya:

Nutrient-dense: High in vitamin C, vitamin A, and folate, papaya supports healthy bones and general wellbeing.

8. Melons (Cantaloupe, Honeydew):

Nutrients: Melons improve bone health and hydration by providing vitamin C, vitamin A, and potassium.

Produce:

• Leafy greens, such as kale, spinach, and collard greens: o Nutrient-dense: high in calcium, vitamin K, and magnesium, which are vital for strong and healthy bones.

• Broccoli:

Nutrients: Calcium, vitamin K, and vitamin C are found in broccoli, which support healthy bones and a strong immune system.

• Brussels Sprouts:

Nutrients: Vitamin K, vitamin C, and folate are found in Brussels sprouts, which promote healthy bones and general nutrition.

• Cabbage:

Nutrients: Vitamin K, vitamin C, and minerals like manganese are found in cabbage, which helps maintain healthy bones.

• **Bell Peppers:**

Nutrients: Vitamin C-rich bell peppers, particularly the red varieties, support the synthesis of collagen for strong bones.

• **Tomatoes:**

Nutrients: Lycopene, potassium, and vitamin C are found in tomatoes and may be beneficial to bone health.

• **Carrots:**

Nutrients: Vitamin A is found in carrots and is necessary for the development and upkeep of bones.

• **Sweet Potatoes:**

Nutrients: High in potassium, manganese, and vitamin A, sweet potatoes promote bone health and general nutrition.

• **Asparagus:**

Nutrients: Vitamin K, vitamin C, and folate are found in asparagus, which supports healthy bones and general wellbeing.

- **Cauliflower:**

Nutrients: Cauliflower supports immune system and bone health by supplying vitamins K, C, and manganese.

A well-rounded intake of nutrients that promote bone health can be achieved by include a range of these fruits and vegetables in your diet. Along with contributing to a balanced and nutrient-dense diet, combining them with other foods high in nutrients helps bone health overall.

Foods to Refrain from or Reduce

It's crucial for people with bone cancer or those who are worried about their bone health to be aware of specific foods that could harm their bone health or make possible side effects from cancer therapies worse. These foods should be limited or avoided:

1. High-Sodium Foods:

• The reason for this is that consuming too much sodium might cause the bones to lose calcium.

• **Foods to Avoid:** restaurant-prepared dishes, processed foods, canned soups, salty snacks, and fast food.

2. Caffeine:

• **Cause:** Excessive caffeine use may hinder the absorption of calcium and cause bone loss.

• **Foods to Avoid:** caffeinated sodas, tea, coffee, and energy drinks.

3. Alcohol:

• **Cause:** Drinking too much alcohol can affect how well calcium is absorbed and cause bone loss.

• **Foods to Avoid:** Beverages with alcohol.

4. High-Phosphorus Foods:

• The reason is that too much phosphorus in comparison to calcium might be harmful to bone health.

• **Foods to Avoid:** Certain packaged foods that include additives, carbonated beverages, and processed meats.

5. High-Sugar Foods:

• **Cause:** Diets heavy in added sugars have the potential to cause inflammation, which may have an impact on bone health.

• **Foods to Avoid:** Candies, sugar-filled snacks, drinks with added sweetness, and desserts.

6. Red and Processed Meats:

• The reason is that consuming large amounts of red and processed meats has been linked to a higher risk of developing several types of cancer.

• Avoid foods like hot dogs, sausages, bacon, and other processed meats. Red meats ought to be eaten sparingly.

7. Fried and High-Fat Foods:

• Theoretically, diets heavy in trans and saturated fats might aggravate inflammation.

• **Foods to Avoid:** processed snacks, fried foods, fast food, and foods with a lot of added fat.

8. High-Oxalate meals:

• **Cause:** High-oxalate meals can exacerbate kidney stone formation, which can be problematic for those with certain forms of bone cancer or renal problems brought on by treatment.

- Avoid foods like spinach, beets, chocolate, almonds, and tea.

9. Over dosage of Vitamin A:

- The rationale is that an excess of vitamin A from supplements may have an adverse effect on bone health.

- **Items to Avoid:** Excessive amounts of vitamin A pills. Make sure you get your vitamin A from whole foods.

It's crucial to remember that each person may react differently to different meals, thus dietary advice should be tailored to the specific person's tastes, treatment plan, and state of health. Always seek the opinion of medical specialists, such as certified dietitians and oncologists, to receive customized counsel and direction based on unique requirements and situations.

Sustaining Optimal Nutritional Balance throughout Therapy

Sustaining general health, controlling side effects, and expediting recovery all depend on maintaining nutritional balance during bone cancer treatment. During treatment, the following tactics can be used to help establish and preserve nutritional balance:

1.   Consulting with medical specialists:

• **Certified Nutritionist/Dietitian:** Collaborate closely with an oncology-focused registered dietitian or nutritionist to obtain individualized food recommendations catered to your unique requirements and course of treatment.

2.   Consistent observation and evaluation:

• **Status Nutritional:** Keep an eye on your nutritional status on a regular basis to spot any deficits or dietary demands changes.

- **Modifications:** Adapt the food plan in light of side effects, overall health, and treatment responses.

3. Sufficient Consumption of Protein:

- **Lean Protein Sources:** To aid in tissue preservation and regeneration, incorporate lean protein sources such fish, chicken, tofu, lentils, and dairy products.

4. A Diet Rich in Nutrients and Balanced:

- **Diversity:** To gain a wide range of vital nutrients, eat a variety of nutrient-dense foods such as fruits, vegetables, whole grains, lean meats, and healthy fats.

5. Hydration:

• **Sufficient Fluid Intake:** Maintain a healthy fluid intake to promote general health and control any possible adverse effects, such as weariness, nausea, and constipation.

6. Calcium and Vitamin D supplementing:

• **Consultation:** Talk to medical specialists about supplementing if you have concerns about obtaining your recommended daily intake of calcium and vitamin D from food.

7. Fiber Intake: To promote digestive health and ward off constipation, eat a diet high in whole grains, fruits, vegetables, and legumes, among other fiber-rich foods.

8. Handling therapy adverse Effects:

• **Texture Adjustments:** Make dietary texture changes in response to adverse effects associated with the therapy (e.g., choosing softer meals if experiencing difficulties swallowing).

• Take into account dietary sensitivities and preferences when adjusting food temperatures (e.g., ingesting cooler foods if experiencing mouth sores).

9. Light Dinners Often:

• **Energy Levels:** To preserve energy levels and control any nausea or fluctuations in appetite, choose modest, frequent meals and snacks.

10. Supplementation as Needed:

• **Consultation:** Seek medical advice before taking supplements if there are particular nutrient shortages or difficulties satisfying dietary requirements just via food.

11. Mindful Eating:

• **Enjoyment of Food:** Develop a positive relationship with food and improve your enjoyment of meals by practicing mindful eating.

12. Customized Approach:

• **Tastes and Tolerances:** To make the diet more sustainable, adjust it to each person's tastes, tolerances, and cultural needs.

13. Frequent Exercise: To promote general well-being, participate in regular, appropriate physical activity based on energy levels and treatment recommendations.

14. Psychosocial Assistance:

• Using a holistic approach, take into account the psychological and emotional elements of diet while undergoing treatment, and seek out psychosocial assistance as required.

15. Honest Communication with Healthcare Team:

• **Side Effect Management:** Share information freely with the healthcare team regarding any side effects of the treatment that may have an impact on eating preferences, dietary practices, or nutritional status.

16. Exercise Caution while Using Supplements:

• **Consultation:** Refrain from using supplements excessively without first seeing medical specialists, as some supplements may interfere with drugs or have detrimental effects on health.

17. Collaborative Approach:

• **Multidisciplinary Team:** For comprehensive care, work with a multidisciplinary healthcare team that includes nurses, nutritionists, oncologists, and other specialists.

Through individualized and comprehensive nutrition during

bone cancer therapy, patients can improve their overall quality of life, maximize their nutritional status, and manage treatment-related problems. Always seek the advice of medical specialists for specific recommendations based on your own requirements and circumstances.

Recipes for a Bone Cancer Diet

When designing recipes for a bone cancer diet, it's important to focus on nutrient-dense ingredients that provide essential vitamins and minerals for bone health. Here are a few recipes that incorporate foods rich in calcium, vitamin D, protein, and other bone-boosting nutrients:

1. Bowl with Salmon and Quinoa: Ingredients:

- **Salmon fillets baked or grilled**
- Cooked quinoa
- Steam-cooked broccoli
- Avocado Slices

- Rosy Tomatoes
- Juice from lemons
- Olive oil
- Fresh Herbs, Like Parsley Or Dill

Guidelines:

1. Place cooked quinoa in a foundation arrangement.
2. Add baked or grilled salmon on top.
3. Add cherry tomatoes, diced avocado, and steaming broccoli.
4. Squeeze in some fresh lemon juice, drizzle with olive oil, and top with fresh herbs.

2. Lentil and Veggie Soup:
Ingredients:

- cooked brown lentils
- chopped carrots
- chopped celery
- chopped spinach or kale
- reduced-sodium vegetable stock
- minced garlic
- Diced onion
- For more flavor, add cumin and turmeric.
- To taste, add salt and pepper.

Directions: Sauté the garlic and onions in a saucepan until aromatic.

1. Add the lentils, celery, and diced carrots.

2. Add the veggie broth with low sodium.

3. Add salt, pepper, cumin, and turmeric for seasoning.

4. Cook until the lentils and veggies are soft.

5. Before serving, stir in chopped kale or spinach.

3. Greek Yogurt Parfait:

Ingredients:

- Unsweetened Greek yogurt
- Berries in season (strawberries, blueberries)
- Chia seeds

- Chopped almonds; optional honey or maple syrup

Instructions:

1. Layer Greek yogurt in a glass or bowl.
2. Top with some delicious berries.
3. Add chopped almonds and chia seeds.
4. If desired, drizzle with maple syrup or honey.

4. Chickpea with Sweet Potato Buddha Bowl:

Ingredients:

- Cubed sweet potatoes that have been roasted
- Chickpeas, roasted
- cooked quinoa
- Raw or sautéed spinach or kale
- Dressing with tahini
- Slices of lemon

Guidelines:

1. For the base, assemble the cooked quinoa.
2. Add roasted chickpeas and sweet potatoes on top.
3. Add some fresh kale or spinach.

4. Pour over some tahini dressing.

5. Accompany with wedges of lemon.

5. Smoothie with Berries and Spinach:

Components:

- A little handful of spinach
- Strawberries, blueberries, and raspberries are mixed berries.
- Greek yogurt without added sugar
- Almond milk or your favorite type of milk
- Chia seeds

- Cubes of ice

- Maple syrup or honey (optional)

Directions: Blend spinach, ice cubes, Greek yogurt, mixed berries, and almond milk until smooth.

1. Add the chia seeds to add some texture.
2. If desired, sweeten with honey or maple syrup.

6. Broccoli with Cauliflower Stir-Fry: Components:

- Florets of cauliflower

- Florets of broccoli

- Cubes of tofu

- Salt-free soy sauce

- minced garlic and ginger
- oil from sesame
- Cooked brown rice

Directions: Stir-fry broccoli, cauliflower, and tofu in sesame oil.

Add the minced garlic and ginger.

Add low-sodium soy sauce and stir to coat the vegetables and tofu.

Place on top of warm brown rice.

Advice:

Control of Portion: Take note of serving amounts to accommodate different dietary requirements.

Hydration: To stay hydrated, drink water or herbal teas with your meals.

Personal Preferences: Adjust recipes to suit dietary restrictions and personal preferences.

It's important to remember to speak with medical specialists, particularly a certified dietitian, to make sure that these recipes meet your unique nutritional requirements while receiving treatment for bone cancer. As necessary, modify the ingredients or preparation techniques in accordance with personal preferences and treatment-related factors.

Exercise and the Risk of Bone Cancer

For those who have bone cancer, physical activity can improve their overall health and quality of life. But considering the particular difficulties and factors related to bone cancer, it's imperative to approach physical activity with prudence and after consulting with medical experts. The following are important things to think about in relation to exercise and bone cancer:

1. Tailored Method:

• Speak with the medical staff: See your healthcare team, including physical therapists and oncologists, before beginning any physical activity to evaluate your specific condition, treatment plan, and any potential limits.

2. Comparing Early and Advanced Stages:

• **Early Stage:** Gradual, low-impact exercise may help people with early-stage bone cancer improve their strength and mobility, particularly following surgery.

- **Advanced Stage:** Individuals at this stage may need to concentrate on activities and motions that are light enough to preserve functionality without placing undue strain on the bones.

3. Low-Impact Exercises:

- **Walking:** This low-impact activity can be modified to suit each person's energy level and level of mobility.

- **Swimming:** By providing buoyancy, swimming or water aerobics lessen the strain on joints.

- **Riding:** One low-impact activity is stationary or recumbent riding.

4. Strength Training:

- **Professional Guidance:** A licensed physical therapist or rehabilitation expert should supervise the performance of strength training exercises.

- **Pay Attention to Core Strength:** Exercises that strengthen the core can enhance stability and assist general function.

5. Stretching and Flexibility:

- **Gentle Stretching:** To increase flexibility, use mild stretching activities.

• **Yoga and Tai Chi:** These forms of exercise place an emphasis on flexibility, balance, and soft motions.

6. Balance Activities:

• **Balance Training:** Use balance drills to lower your chance of falling, particularly if your bone density is weak.

• **Easy Balance Drills:** Practice heel-to-toe walking, stand on one leg, and utilize stability aids as necessary.

7. Modifications for Adverse Reactions to Treatment:

- **Fatigue:** Take into account brief, frequent sessions and modify exercise levels according to energy levels.

- **Bone Pain:** If you have bone pain, try to limit your activity and concentrate on making soft movements.

- **Weight-Bearing Exercise:** Depending on the location and severity of their bone cancer, some people may need to refrain from performing weight-bearing exercises.

8.   Observation   and correspondence:

•   **Frequent   Check-Ins:** Communicate any changes in physical activity and address any concerns by scheduling regular check-ins with your healthcare team.

• **Open Communication:** Discuss any pain, discomfort, or difficulties you may be having while engaging in physical exercise.

9. Psychosocial Advantages:

• **Emotional Well-Being:** Engaging in physical activity can help elevate mood, lessen stress, and improve general wellbeing.

- **Support Groups:** Take into account participating in activities that promote social relationships and emotional support, as well as joining support groups.

10. Modified Tools and Methods:

- **Assistive Devices:** To promote safe and efficient movement, take into account the use of adapted equipment or assistive devices, depending on individual needs.

- **Activity Modification:** Adapt workouts to specific situations, such as using a chair for sitting exercises.

11. Steer clear of risky activities:

• **Contact Sports**: Steer clear of contact and high-impact sports that could injure your weakened bones.

• **Extreme Activities:** Avoid engaging in any activity that puts you at danger of fractures or falls.

12. Consistent observation and modification:

• **Consult the medical staff:** Consult your medical team on a regular basis to evaluate your physical state and modify your exercise regimen as necessary.

Safety should always come first, and you should be honest with your healthcare provider about any worries or modifications to your physical activity schedule. Finding a balance that enhances general wellbeing and helps your unique treatment plan is the aim.

Conclusion

To sum up, bone cancer is a difficult and complex illness that calls for a multifaceted strategy that includes medical care, dietary assistance, and deliberate physical exercise. Patients with bone cancer must collaborate closely with their oncologists, dietitians, and physical therapists to create a customized treatment plan that takes into account their individual needs and circumstances.

• Knowledge of the different forms, causes, risk factors, symptoms, and diagnosis is essential to understanding bone cancer. A well-balanced diet rich in important nutrients is essential for maintaining bone health throughout cancer therapy. Nutrition plays a critical role in this regard. A range of foods high in calcium, vitamin D, protein, and other nutrients that support bone health should be included, although dietary restrictions and treatment-related adverse effects should be considered as well.

• When done carefully and under the direction of medical specialists, physical activity can improve strength, mobility, and general well-being. Exercises for balance, flexibility, and low-impact aerobics that are customized for each person's skills can be helpful. But it's important to modify exercise regimens according to cancer stage, side effects of medication, and personal tolerances.

• Sustaining nutritional equilibrium while undergoing therapy necessitates consistent observation, modifications according to treatment outcomes, and a customized strategy. Key factors for a well-rounded approach to diet are minimizing treatment-related adverse effects, increasing protein consumption, and staying hydrated.

It's crucial to eat a range of nutrient-dense foods throughout bone cancer treatment in terms of nutrition. Fruits, vegetables, whole grains, lean meats, and sources of vital vitamins and minerals are all included in this. Furthermore, limiting or avoiding certain foods, such as those heavy in sugar and sodium, can improve general health.

Bone cancer diet recipes ought to emphasize the use of nutrient-dense ingredients and be flexible enough to accommodate dietary restrictions and personal tastes. To promote general health, these dishes may contain a range of proteins, whole grains, fruits, and vegetables.

The treatment of bone cancer necessitates a team effort that is holistic in nature, considering the mental, physical, and nutritional dimensions of health. Navigating this difficult disease requires a strong support network, consistent communication with healthcare providers, and a dedication to self-care.

It's critical to keep in mind that the information offered here is generic in nature. Individualized advice from medical specialists is essential for developing a customized plan that addresses the particular requirements of each person diagnosed with bone cancer.

THE END